DIABETES EPIDEMIC, WHICH IS ON THE RISE

Best Foods For Diabetes Management

By

Dr. Jacob D. Byrne

Content

Introduction

Diabetes is also known as diabetes mellitus, and it can be roughly categorized as a group of illnesses when a person has excessive blood sugar levels. This could be due to either insufficient insulin synthesis or a failure on the part of the body to react to the insulin appropriately. Some of the signs and symptoms of diabetes include frequent hunger, thirst, and urination.

Diabetes is sometimes a chronic disorder marked by elevated blood glucose levels.

The disorder affects 382 million people worldwide and is a common one. As of 2013, there were 382 million people worldwide who were affected by the disorder.

Chapter 1

Type 1 and Type 2 Diabetes

Type 1 and Type 2 diabetes are the two most common classifications for diabetes. When a person has type 1 diabetes, their body stops producing insulin. Only 10% of those who have the disease suffer from Type 1 diabetes, which is also sometimes called insulin-dependent diabetes or early onset diabetes. This kind of diabetes is quite exceptional.

And this type of diabetes is more common in persons under 40, even in adolescence or the early stages of adulthood.

A person with type 1 diabetes must take insulin injections for the rest of their lives, adhere to a strict diet, and regularly get blood tests to check their blood glucose levels.

However, type 2 diabetes is much more common than type 1 diabetes, and over 90% of those who have this illness have type 2 diabetes.

Insulin resistance, a disease associated with type 2 diabetes, occurs when the body does not create enough insulin or when the body cells do not respond to insulin.

For many people, type 2 diabetes is a condition that is relatively easier to manage. One can prevent type 2 diabetes symptoms by keeping their weight within healthy ranges, eating a healthy diet, exercising regularly, and monitoring their blood sugar levels frequently.

Obstetric Diabetes

Gestational diabetes, which is a type of diabetes that affects pregnant women, is a significant classification of the disease.

Sometimes during pregnancy, women have blood sugar levels that are on the higher side, and their bodies don't create enough insulin to carry this glucose into their cells.

Only during pregnancy can gestational diabetes be diagnosed, and the vast majority of people can manage their disease with diet and exercise. However, 10–20% of individuals require the use of particular drugs to maintain control of their blood glucose levels.

Making sure to eat a low-cholesterol diet when pregnant is a crucial step in helping someone prevent the illness.

What Causes Diabetes in People?

When someone is overweight, they have a greater chance of getting diabetes. One of the causes of the same is that when someone is fat, their body generates chemicals that might contribute to the destabilization of their cardiovascular and metabolic systems.

Therefore, having type 2 diabetes, being overweight, and eating the wrong kind

of diet are all associated. Aging is a significant factor that is known to significantly increase the risk of having type 2 diabetes.

Alternately, some of the additional risk factors for diabetes include genetics, family history, or even adhering to a poor eating plan.

Chapter 2

Diabetes Risk Assessment

A study published in the Lancet, a major international medical publication, in August 2014 discovered that the risk of having diabetes among Americans is quickly growing.

The study also discovered that your risk depends on your race, education, and where you live and that diabetics live longer lives.

This is the first study in more than a decade to calculate the risk of acquiring diabetes in Americans. It was carried out by epidemiologists at

the US Centers for Disease Control and Prevention in Atlanta, Georgia, who have been following and studying diabetes prevalence and the rate at which new cases are identified for many years.

The researchers analyzed mortality data for over 600,000 people from 1985 to 2011 (25 years) to determine the likelihood of having type 1 or type 2 diabetes (excluding gestational diabetes).

Though the study only looked at diabetes in the context of Americans, identical results would likely have been found if the study had been undertaken using European data or data from other nations where a

Western-style diet and lifestyle are the norm.

The ever-increasing danger of diabetes According to the study, there was a substantial increase in the overall probability that an American will develop diabetes between 1985 and 2011.

In 1985, American boys had a 21% likelihood of having diabetes, while girls had a 27% chance. By 2011, however, that risk had risen to 40% for both boys and girls. In other words, the risk for boys had nearly doubled, while the risk for girls had increased by 50%.

The Lancet study did not investigate why this is so. However, one reason

could be that individuals are living longer lives, giving them more years in which to develop diabetes.

Diabetics are living longer lives.

The good news is that American children with diabetes can now expect to live for more than 70 years.

Indeed, between 1985 and 2011, the number of years that males diagnosed with diabetes might anticipate life grew by 156%. For women, the figure was 70%. Though the researchers provided no reason, this is most likely owing to developments in medical knowledge and therapies over the last 25 years.

Being diabetic reduces your life expectancy. Over the 25-year study period, the average number of years lost owing to diabetes for the population grew by 46 percent in men and 44 percent in women. This is attributable to the rising prevalence of diabetes. It could also be attributable to the fact that there are fewer undetected instances currently. While the overall picture appears to be getting bleaker, things are looking up for the individual diabetic.

Between the 1990s and the end of the 2000s, the number of years of life a man diagnosed with diabetes can anticipate loss fell by about two years (from 7.7 to 5.8 lost years).

Women gained an average of two years (their losses dropping from 8.7 to 6.8 years) throughout the same period. These advancements are most likely the result of improved treatment regimens.

Diabetes, race, and gender

While most Americans have a 40 percent probability of developing diabetes, the picture for Blacks and Hispanics is far worse.

Diabetes is 37% more likely in white boys than in white girls. By contrast, the possibilities for Black men are 44.7%, while the risk for their sisters is a whopping 55.3%. Hispanic boys and girls have a 51.8% and 51.5% likelihood of having diabetes, respectively.

These numbers, which allude to the risks of having diabetes, support the notion that diabetes has a hereditary origin, at least to the extent that your genes can predispose you to diabetes. Most medical researchers think that it is your lifestyle that sets it in motion.

According to the researchers, they investigated race because that was the data they had available; however, they did acknowledge that socioeconomic class is likely as relevant as, if not more important than, race.

Nonetheless, Whites have a lower risk of having diabetes than Blacks and Hispanics. Indeed, the risk for White girls is one-third that of Black and Hispanic women.

As you can see, Hispanics of both sexes, as well as Black women, have a risk that exceeds 50%.
But genetic differences cannot explain why Black men have a risk that is around 10 percentage points lower than Black women.

Diabetes and education

The less educated you are, the more likely you are to get diabetes.
According to the Lancet, the frequency of new illnesses among high-school dropouts was 6.5 per thousand in 1990, 3.6 among high-school graduates, and 3.2 among those who studied beyond high school.

This figure represents the number of new diabetes diagnoses among high-school dropouts, high-school graduates, and those who continued to study after high school. In 2008 it

peaked at 15.6, 9.4, and 6.5 percent per thousand, respectively.

Since then, the rate at which new diagnoses are discovered has slowed slightly. This could be attributed to bettering lives.
At the same time, according to the most recent statistics, high-school dropouts are twice as likely as those who continued their education after graduating from high school to get diabetes.

It appears that the more educated you are, the more likely you are to live a healthy lifestyle and take the threat of diabetes seriously.

Where you live and diabetes The risk of having diabetes appears to vary from state to state in the United States.

Diabetes affects 11.7 percent of the population of Mississippi, for example. This figure is 11.5 percent in Louisiana. In South Dakota and Hawaii, by contrast, only 7% of the population is diabetic.

The percentage of people with diabetes in the other states of the Union ranges from 7 to 11.7 percent.

What causes these variances are unknown, but it is likely a combination of education, dietary cultures, exercise habits, and genetics. Climate may also play a role, however, this has not been researched as far as I am aware.

THE IMPLICATION

Continual increases in the number of new instances of diabetes identified each year, combined with longer life expectancy, have increased the risk of having diabetes as well as the number of years spent coping with the condition. At the same time, the

average person is losing fewer years of his or her life owing to the disease. The Lancet study's findings indicate that there will be a continuing need for health services and considerable expenditure to control the disease. They also underline the need for effective treatments to lower the occurrence of diabetes, such as healthy lifestyle education and regular testing of the entire community to detect pre-diabetes.

Is it possible to reverse diabetes?

Brown rice is an excellent choice for those seeking an unconventional way to naturally cure diabetes.

Yes, researchers at Harvard University recently examined brown rice in a big study sample.

Three studies including approximately 40,000 men and over 150,000 women discovered that eating brown rice twice a week reduces the risk of type 2 diabetes by 11%.

Simple common sense tactics are the most effective way to reduce the effects of this condition and, in the long term, maybe eliminate the need for insulin injections.

Chapter 3

Diabetes-Friendly Foods

Te food you eat is one of the things that can get you into difficulties with diabetes. If you have diabetes or are pre-diabetic, one way to cure, control, or avoid diabetes is to focus on foods that can help cure or reduce your chance of acquiring the chronic condition. It may appear to be a Herculean undertaking to try to change your eating habits since, let's face it, many bad things are uite tasty. Regardless, you can make a difference. Some of the best diabetic foods are also delicious.

Before considering the best meals for diabetics, consider the type of diabetes you have as well as the goals you want to achieve by making dietary modifications.

Type I diabetes is not prevented, cannot be cured and necessitates daily insulin injections. Using food to control type 1 diabetes is done to ensure that complications, both long and short-term, are reduced by normalizing blood glucose levels with the use of diet.

Type II diabetes, on the other hand, can not only be prevented, but in some circumstances cured, or the patient's dependency on drugs or insulin injections can be greatly decreased.

Making dietary changes for type II diabetes (and increasing daily physical activity levels) has the goal of assisting with weight loss and assisting the patient in maintaining normal body weight. While the causes of type II diabetes vary, being overweight or obese is one key factor

that raises the risk of having type 2 diabetes.

Diabetic Friendly Foods

(1) Carbohydrates

The body requires carbs that it converts into glucose, which is the source of energy or fuel required by the body's cells. Carbohydrates are found in almost all diets, except meat, poultry, and fish.

The two types of carbohydrates used by the body are generated from complex carbs (starches) such as beans, pasta, rice, and so on. The second form of carbohydrate is

known as simple carbs, which refer to sugars obtained from fruits, vegetables, honey, white table sugar, and so on.

If you have diabetes, you should learn about carbohydrates. Diabetics should eat a diet rich in carbs, particularly complex carbohydrates, rather than any other form of food. Simple carbs raise blood sugar levels faster than complex carbohydrates (grains, beans, peas, peanuts, soybeans, potatoes, and so on), which raise blood sugar levels slowly.

Simple carbs may not be fully off limits for diabetics, but this is something to address with your doctor because many "forbidden

items," such as white table sugar, may not be completely off limits.

Carbohydrate counting is probably a good idea for every diabetic. Following a talk with your doctor about how You can then pick how many carbs you need in a day and what your daily carb mix will be. You may then be able to have a candy bar here, as long as you consider how much the candy bar will affect your daily permissible carbohydrate intake.
requirements in the same way that you would consider a cup of beans, a cup of pasta, etc.

2. Fiber

The reason that complex carbs and whole grains are important for diabetics is because of the fiber content, which is why refined "foods" are strictly forbidden for diabetics because they are stripped of fiber and raise blood sugar levels very quickly because foods are digested very quickly when they lack fiber.

Fiber has numerous health benefits, including alleviating constipation, lowering the risk of heart disease, lowering cholesterol, and aiding in weight loss. Fiber-rich foods are one of the best foods for diabetics since fiber can help control blood sugar levels, so adopting a fiber-rich diet is a must for everyone who wants to overcome or prevent diabetes.

There are two forms of fiber, and each is very significant. The first type is known as soluble fiber, while the second is known as insoluble fiber.

Soluble fiber

Soluble fiber, which is found mostly in beans, oats, some fruits and vegetables, and so on, dissolves in water and forms a gel in the stomach. The sticky nature of insoluble fiber aids in slowing digestion. This slowing down helps to minimize blood sugar spikes, which is a very strong role in diabetes cure or control, and it also helps to regulate blood sugar levels by avoiding glucose from being consumed too instantly into the blood.

Spikes in blood sugar levels indicate that there will be an excess of glucose in the blood, which the body may have difficulty transporting to or storing, which could lead to difficulties and, in extreme cases, death.

Another advantage of soluble fiber is that if you have insulin resistance, which is a common feature of type 2 diabetes development, soluble fiber can help to increase the sensitivity of the body's cells to insulin, allowing the insulin to remove more glucose from the blood and distribute it to the various cells in the body.

Insoluble fiber

Insoluble fiber does not dissolve in water and hence travels through the body intact, aiding in the flow of food through the intestines and thereby preventing constipation.

The insoluble fiber found mostly in wheat, as well as certain fruits and vegetables, has been associated with a lower risk of diabetes.

Several studies have indicated that those who eat fiber-rich (or complex carbohydrate-rich) diets were able to reach and maintain normal blood sugar levels by as much as 90% for those with type 2 diabetes and 30% for those with type 1 diabetes.

An important aspect of a high fiber diet is to boost your water intake. Fiber requires a large amount of water to flow through the body and do what it needs to do. Increasing your water intake can also keep you hydrated, which is vital for your overall health and well-being.

Consuming more fiber is also a fantastic way to avoid acquiring diabetes if you have already been classified as pre-diabetic.

3. Beneficial fats

There are no two diabetes diets that are the same. While one diabetic may be encouraged to consume less fat, another may be urged to consume more fats (the healthy kind).

The amount of healthy fat content is something to discuss with your doctor, but it has been discovered that some people who eat less healthy fats and more carbohydrates may unwittingly increase their levels of triglycerides in their bodies, which has been linked to a higher risk of heart disease in diabetics.

This is because, when compared to carbs, fat and protein do not elevate blood sugar levels as quickly, and this helps to lower triglyceride levels.

If this is a problem for you, increasing your consumption of healthy fats such as olive oil will not only lower your blood sugar levels but will also minimize your risk of heart disease. Decent fats, such as those based on olive oil, avocados,

and numerous nuts, are also high in antioxidants, which are beneficial for diabetes management and will be addressed further below.

4. Minerals and vitamins

Many issues can occur from diabetes that can impact the nerves, eyes, blood vessels, and so on, and some vitamins can help promote healthy eyes, blood vessels, nerves, and so on. Foods containing vitamins C and E, as well as the mineral zinc, are among the best foods for diabetes.

These vitamins and minerals are known as antioxidants because they help to prevent free radical damage

to the body's cells. Free radical damage to cells can raise the likelihood of developing diabetes-related problems such as nerve damage and heart disease. Antioxidants aid in the protection of cells from free radicals.

Many diabetics have been discovered to be magnesium deficient, which can raise the risk of diabetes-related eye disorders as well as heart disease. Magnesium insufficiency has been related to retina damage, thus boosting your magnesium intake will help protect your eyes and heart from any consequences.

Another mineral that many diabetics are lacking in is chromium. Chromium is significant because it

can help the body manage blood sugar levels better. This mineral can be found in broccoli, fortified breakfast cereals, grapefruit, and other foods.
Vitamin and mineral shortages are frequent in diabetics, so if you aren't getting enough of these elements from your diet, a decent supplement may help.

Finding a meal plan that works for you that mixes these many ingredients - fiber, vitamins, minerals, fats, etc - to help control blood sugar levels either directly or indirectly is an important feature of using food to treat, and manage, or prevent diabetes healthily.

Chapter 4

Diabetes home remedies

Diabetes is manageable if you are committed to your health.
Plan your routine and nutrition, and you'll be astonished at how easy diabetes management may be.

1. Coriander, cucumber, cabbage, coconut, chenopodium album, pumpkin creeper, cucumber, cabbage, bitter guard, carrot, tomato, lemon, radish, onion, and ginger are all excellent choices.

2. Eat fiber-rich foods like apples, figs, guava, lemon, and orange.
Fiber grains include barley, oats, maize, wheat flour, sorghum, pearl millet, whole wheat, rice flakes, refined wheat flour (without husk), and puffed rice.
Fiber-rich foods include coriander seeds, cumin seeds, dried pepper, and turmeric.

3. Wet 90-100 seeds in 250 gms of water at night.
Mash them in the morning, strain through a cloth, and drink the concoction daily.
To get rid of diabetes, take it twice a day for two months.

4. To naturally treat diabetes, combine equal parts bael and parijat leaf juice.
Grab two teaspoons of it two times a day.
5. Eat grapefruits daily as a natural diabetic treatment.

www.ingramcontent.com/pod-product-compliance
Lightning Source LLC
LaVergne TN
LVHW020532160826
845677LV00015B/4021

* 9 7 9 8 8 4 6 0 9 5 3 6 6 *